The Unofficial
Plant Paradox
Cookbook

Low-Lectin Lifestyle

69 FAN-BASED RECIPES INSPIRED BY THE PLANT PARADOX

Note to Readers:

This is a summary and analysis companion book based on The Plant Paradox: The Hidden Dangers in "Healthy" Foods That Cause Disease and Weight Gain by Steven R. Gundry M.D. It is meant to enhance your original reading experience, but is not meant to supplement the entire book.

We strongly recommend you pick up the original book, along with Gundry's awesome authorized cookbook as well.

Table of Contents

Introduction

This collection of recipes is intended to help you incorporate a low-lectin diet into your lifestyle. It will briefly outline the basics ideas behind the diet and what foods eat and which to avoid.

A low-lectin diet does not have to be a boring one. The recipes in this volume will show that a low-lectin lifestyle can be fun and versatile. The low-lectin diet is becoming increasingly popular and you will find a number of websites dedicated to providing recipes and tips for reducing your lectin intake. With a low-lectin diet, the only limiting thing is your imagination.

Lectins?

The Low-Lectin Diet is based on research conducted and published by Dr. Stephen Gundry. In his New York Times Best Selling book 'The Plant Paradox: The Hidden Dangers in "Healthy" Foods that Cause Disease and Weight Gain,' Dr. Gundry outlines how decades of research have led him to believe that some of the most common foods we eat contain proteins harmful to humans.

Lectins are large proteins present in many plants that have evolved over millennia as a defense mechanism to protect themselves and their seeds from animal predators. We are all aware of one of the most famous lectins: gluten. These proteins bind to molecules, including sugar, earning them the nickname "sticky proteins." This binding can interrupt messaging between cells and cause toxic and inflammatory reactions.

The problem of harmful lectins extends to the meat we eat. Grain- or soy-fed beef and poultry causes problems for humans who consume them and their products, such as eggs, milk, and cheese.

Lectins found in **beans**, **legumes**, **nightshades**, traditional **dairy** products, **seeds**, and **grain-fed animal proteins** should be avoided. The next couple pages will provide a list of products you should eat.

Remember to be creative and have fun!

Symptoms of Lectins:

- Brain fog
- Allergies
- Stubborn weight gain
- Aches and pains
- Acid reflux disease
- Acne
- Diabetes
- Depression
- Hypertension
- Irritable Bowel Syndrome
- Chronic fatigue
- Asthma
- Canker sores
- Hearth disease
- Hypertension
- Peripheral neuropathy
- Vitiligo

For a complete list, see: The Plant Paradox – Patterns Causing Problems.

What To Eat

Oils
Algae oil
Olive oil
Coconut oil
Macadamia oil
Avocado oil
Walnut oil
Red palm
Rice bran
Sesame oil

Sweeteners
Stevia
Just Like Sugar
Inulin
Yacon
Monk fruit
Xylitol

Nuts and Seeds
Macadamia
Walnuts
Pistachios
Pecans
Coconut
Hazelnuts
Chestnuts
Brazil nuts
Flaxseeds
Hemp seeds
Psyllium

Olives
All

Chocolate
72% or greater cocoa

Vinegars
All

Herbs and Seasonings
All
Miso

Flours
Coconut
Almond
Hazelnut
Sesame
Chestnut
Cassava
Arrowroot
Grape seed
Tiger nut
Sweet potato
Green banana

Noodles and Rice
Cappelo's fetuccine
Pasta Slim
Shirataki noodles
Kelp noodles
Miracle noodles
Miracle rice

'Dairy' Products
Coconut milk
Coconut cream
French/Italian Butter
Buffalo butter
Ghee
Goat milk yogurt
Coconut yogurt
Sheep cheese and yogurt
Goat and sheep kefir
Parmesan
French and Italian cheese

Swiss cheese
Buffalo mozzarella
Heavy cream
Organic sour cream
Casein A-2 milk

Fish (wild only)
Whitefish
Bass
Canned tuna
Salmon
Halibut
Shrimp
Crab
Lobster
Scallops
Squid
Clams
Oyster
Mussels
Sardines
Anchovies

Fruits (limited, except avocado)
Avocados
All berries
Cherries
Pears
Pomegranates
Kiwis
Apples
Nectarines
Plums
Peaches
Apricots
Figs
Dates

Vegetables
Broccoli
Brussel sprouts
Cauliflower
Bok choy
Cabbage
Swiss chard
Arugula
Watercress
Collards
Kale
Radicchio
Kimchi
Raw sauerkraut
Celery
Onions
Leeks
Chives
Scallions
Carrots
Artichokes
Beets

Radishes
Cilantro
Asparagus
Garlic
Mushrooms
All leafy greens

Starches
Green plantains
Baobab fruit
Cassava
Sweet potatoes, yams
Jicama
Taro root
Green mango
Green papaya
Sorghum

Meat
(free range/grass-fed)
Chicken
Turkey

Ostrich
Duck
Eggs
Goose
Pheasant
Quail
Bison
Wild game
Venison
Boar
Elk
Pork
Lamb
Beef
Prosciutto

Meat Alternatives
Quorn
Hemp tofu
Hiliary's Root
Tempeh

Breakfast

There is lots you can do with breakfast on a low-lectin diet. Get creative with different vegetables and meat alternatives to keep your breakfasts fresh and interesting.

SWISS CHARD OMELETTE
SERVED WITH FRESH FRUIT

Time 10 min | Servings 2-3

This low-lectin breakfast is the perfect start to your day. Ensure you use pasteurized or Omega-3 eggs. If not sharing, store in refrigerator for a ready-to-go breakfast or lunch.

INGREDIENTS

Swiss chard, 1 bunch

5 eggs, large

¼ onion, chopped

4 cloves garlic, crushed

3-4 tbsp. extra-virgin olive oil

pepper, freshly ground

Fresh blueberries or raspberries

DIRECTIONS

In a medium-sized pot, boil water and cook chard until tender. Remove chard, squeezing water from the leaves in handfuls. Pat dry with paper towel.

In a medium-sized bowl, beat eggs and continually mix while adding chard, salt, and pepper.

In a medium-sized skillet, add garlic and onion and cook until the onions are translucent. Remove and discard garlic.

Add the egg mixture to the skillet. Push the cooked outside edges of the egg mixture toward the center, tilting the skillet so the raw egg mixture spreads to the edges.

Reduce heat and cover skillet. Let cook for 2-3 minutes.

With a spatula, fold one half of the omelette over the other. Flip the entire omelette onto its other side. Cook until golden brown on the outside.

Serve with a side of fresh blueberries or raspberries.

TURKEY CHORIZO SCRAMBLED EGGS WITH GOAT CHEESE

Time 10 min | Servings 2

This simple breakfast is easy to make, delicious, and will impress everyone. Consider adding spinach for an even healthier option.

INGREDIENTS

4 eggs, large

½ tbsp. butter, French or Italian

¼ onion, chopped

4-5 button mushrooms, sliced

7-10 slices turkey chorizo

2 tbsp. goat cheese, crumbled

pepper, freshly ground

salt

handful chives, chopped

DIRECTIONS

In a medium-sized skillet, melt butter over medium-high heat and sauté mushrooms and onions. Stir occasionally until onions are translucent.

Beat eggs thoroughly in a medium-sized bowl. Add onions, mushrooms, turkey chorizo, and season with salt and pepper. Mix thoroughly.

Pour mixture into skillet stirring until nearly cooked. Add goat cheese and stir for another 30 seconds.

Garnish with thinly chopped chives.

CINNAMON PANCAKES

Prep 25 min | Servings 4

These cinnamon pancakes are perfect for a comforting morning dish. Avoid using traditional flour sources, instead opt for cassava or arrowroot flour.

INGREDIENTS

1 cup cassava flour

2 tbsp. sweetener

1 tbsp. baking powder

1 tsp. cinnamon

¼ tsp. salt

1/8 tsp. nutmeg

1 ¼ cup goat's milk kefir

½ tsp. vanilla extract

2 eggs, large

3 ½ tbsp. butter, French or Italian

¼ cup water

DIRECTIONS

In a medium-sized skillet, melt ½ tbsp. of butter.

Mix flour, sweetener, baking powder, cinnamon, nutmeg, and salt in a medium-sized bowl.

In a large bowl, mix together eggs, kefir, vanilla, and water until thoroughly mixed. Add butter and mix thoroughly.

Add the flour mixture to the egg mixture; whisk until completely combined.

Pour ¼ cup-sized portions of the batter into the skillet. Let cook until bubbles appear on the surface of the pancake. With a spatula, flip the pancake and cook until golden brown on both sides.

Serve pancakes with a dollop of butter and sprinkled with cinnamon.

Sweeteners
Artificial sweeteners are a disruptive element in our everyday diets. They change your gut microbiome and contribute to weight gain. Avoid Stevia, sucralose, Equal, and aspartame. Try the ones below instead:

- Stevia
- Yacon
- Xylitol

BLUEBERRY BREAKFAST BARS

Prep 25 min | Servings 8-10

These delicious low-lectin breakfast bars are bursting with blueberries and are great option for breakfasts on the go.

INGREDIENTS

1 ½ cups almond flour

2 tbsp. coconut flour

½ tsp. baking soda

¼ tsp. salt

1/2 tsp. cinnamon

¼ cup coconut sugar

3 tbsp. coconut oil

3 eggs

1 tsp. vanilla extract

16 oz. blueberries

DIRECTIONS

Preheat oven to 350 degrees Fahrenheit.

Mix almond flour, coconut flour, baking soda, cinnamon, and salt together in a medium-sized bowl.

In an additional medium-sized bowl, mix together coconut oil, eggs, coconut sugar, and vanilla extract until thoroughly mixed.

Pour the egg mixture into the flour mixture slowly while stirring until completely mixed.

Line an 8x8 baking pan with parchment paper and pour batter into the pan.

Smooth the surface of the batter with a spatula and cover with blueberries, pushing down lightly so they are half deep in batter.

Bake for 20 minutes.

YOGURT, BERRY BREAKFAST BOWL WITH AVOCADO

Prep 5 min | Servings 1

Although light, this breakfast still packs an energy punch. Try using different seasonal berries to keep things fresh.

INGREDIENTS

1 cup coconut yogurt

½ avocado, sliced

1 ½ tbsp. flax seed

handful blueberries

handful raspberries

2-3 leaves fresh mint, chopped

DIRECTIONS

In a medium sized bowl add yogurt and top with flax seed, avocado, mint, and berries.

Berries can be seasonal, including raspberries, blueberries, or blackberries.

YOGURT
Yogurt made from cows contain A1 Casein, a protein which is harmful and should be avoided. This includes Greek yogurt. Safe alternatives include:

- Coconut yogurt
- Goat's milk yogurt
- Buffalo milk yogurt
- Sheep's milk yogurt

SCRAMBLED EGG, GOAT CHEESE BREAKFAST BURRITOS

Prep 25 min | Servings 4

These savory breakfast burritos are sure to be a favorite. Consider preparing in advance and freezing for a quick and portable breakfast on the run.

INGREDIENTS

Tortillas

1 ½ cups cassava flour

1 cup warm water

1/4 cup butter, French or Italian

Burrito filling

2 tbsp. extra-virgin olive oil

2 oz. fresh spinach, chopped

2 cloves garlic, thinly sliced

6 eggs, beaten

4 oz. goat cheese, crumbled

pepper, freshly ground

salt

Variations:
Consider adding organic, ground turkey or chicken to your breakfast burritos.

DIRECTIONS

Melt butter in the microwave in a medium-size, microwave-safe bowl. Whisk melted butter and warm water.

Add flour to the butter mixture and mix into a dough. Keep adding more water or flour until the dough no longer sticks to your hands.

Roll dough into a firm ball. Remove 2.5 oz. sized chunks from the large ball and roll into a smaller ball. Place smaller ball between to sheets of parchment paper and flatten out with a rolling pin.

Preheat non-stick frying-pan to medium-high heat. Do not grease the pan. Carefully place your rolled-out tortilla into the skillet and cook for 90 seconds on each side or until lightly browned.

Burrito filling

In a medium-sized frying-pan, heat oil over medium heat. Cook garlic and spinach until the latter is wilted. Season with salt and pepper. Spread spinach evenly around the bottom of the frying pan.

Beat the eggs in a medium-sized bowl and pour over the spinach and garlic. Continue mixing the eggs and spinach until eggs are almost cooked. Turn off heat and crumble goat cheese evenly over the scrambled eggs and let soften.

Fold egg mixture in microwave-warmed burritos and serve.

SPINACH AND CHEESE QUICHE

Prep 50 min | Servings 4-6

Loaded with the low-lectin spinach, this cheesy, savory dish is perfect for breakfast and afternoon snacks. Refrigerate left-overs for next day's breakfast.

INGREDIENTS

1 tbsp. extra-virgin olive oil

1 onion, chopped

10 oz. fresh spinach, chopped

5 eggs, beaten

2 cups goat cheese, crumbled

1 cup mushrooms, sliced

pepper, freshly ground

salt

DIRECTIONS

Preheat oven to 350 degrees Fahrenheit.

In large frying pan, heat oil on medium-high heat. Add onions. Stir occasionally and cook until onions are clear and soft. Stir in mushrooms and spinach.

In a large bowl, mix eggs, cheese, salt, and pepper. Add spinach and mushroom mixture and stir thoroughly.

Pour mixture into a greased 9-inch pie pan.

Bake in oven for approximately 30 minutes. Let sit and cool for 10 minutes prior to serving.

CHEESE
Cheese made from cows contain A1 Casein, a high-lectin protein which should be avoided. Safe alternatives include:

- Goat cheese (including brie)
- High fat French, Italian or Swiss cheeses
- Buffalo mozzarella

AVOCADO BREAKFAST CUPS

Time 15 min | Servings 2-4

This warm, savory breakfast is quick and easy to make and packed with energy to keep you going all morning long. Consider adding a pinch of paprika for even more flavor.

INGREDIENTS

4 eggs, medium

2 avocados, ripe

1 tbsp. butter

1 sprig thyme

pepper, freshly ground

salt

DIRECTIONS

Preheat oven to 400 degrees Fahrenheit.

Cut and separate each avocado into two halves. Scoop out a small hole in the middle of each half.

Create avocado cups by cracking an egg into each half.

Top each half with butter, thyme, salt, and pepper.

Place in a baking pan and cook for 10 minutes.

BLUEBERRY AVOCADO SUPER SMOOTHIE

Prep 5 min | Servings 1

This smoothie is packed with energy and nutrients for the perfect start to your day. Alternatively, prepare one for your mid-afternoon snack to give you the extra boost to get through your day. Add some protein powder for an extra kick.

INGREDIENTS

1 cup blueberries

1 cup spinach, fresh

½ avocado

1 tbsp. flax seeds

¼ tsp. cinnamon

1 tbsp. organic honey, raw

½ cup ice

mint leaves, fresh

DIRECTIONS

Cut and separate avocado into two halves. Using only one half, remove the pit and skin.

Place all ingredients, minus the mint and a couple blueberries, into the blender. Puree until thoroughly blended and thick in consistency.

Pour into glass and top with blueberries and fresh mint.

Protein Powders
Many soy and whey protein powders are high in lectins. If you're looking for a low-lectin alternative try golden pea protein isolate powder, a high protein, low-lectin supplement perfect for smoothies.

These powders use an enzymatic isolation process which removes lectins, but keeps high levels of protein.

GREEN SMOOTHIE

Prep 5 min | Servings 1-2

This smoothie is full of healthy vegetables and energy. It's also a great pick-me up for the afternoons.

INGREDIENTS

½ cup parsley

½ cup spinach

½ cup kale

1 green apple

½ lemon

½ avocado

2 tsp. ginger, grated

1 cup coconut milk

½ cup ice

DIRECTIONS

Cut and separate avocado into two halves. Using only one half, remove the pit and skin.

Remove move stems from parsley. Peel half a lemon and remove the seeds.

Place all ingredients into blender. Puree until thoroughly blended and thick in consistency.

Pour into glass and serve.

Dressings

The options for salads on a low-lectin diet are endless. The large variety of fresh, organic vegetables and cheeses make finding a healthy meal easy. Pair with the following dressings for a low-lectin, crowd-pleasing meal.

All dressing should be stored in the refrigerator until served. Homemade dressings are good for up to 5 days.

Refer to the 'what to eat' section for which vegetables to include in your next salad.

BASIL VINAGARETTE

INGREDIENTS

1 cup fresh basil

1 clove garlic

1 shallot

½ cup extra-virgin olive oil

2 tbsp. red wine vinegar

½ tsp. red pepper flakes

pepper, freshly ground

salt

DIRECTIONS

Chop shallot and remove stems from the fresh basil leaves.

Combine ingredients in a food processer and blend until smooth. Adjust seasoning as needed.

DAIRY-FREE, CREAMY AVOCADO DRESSING

INGREDIENTS

1 avocado, large

¼ cup extra-virgin olive oil

1 bunch cilantro

2-3 cloves garlic

1 lime

2 tbsp. apple cider vinegar

1 tbsp. honey, raw

¼ cup water

DIRECTIONS

Remove stems from the fresh cilantro leaves.

Combine all ingredients in a food processer and blend until smooth. Adjust seasoning and amount of water as needed.

CREAMY DILL DRESSING

INGREDIENTS

½ cup coconut milk yogurt

¼ cup homemade mayonnaise

1 tsp. dill, dried

1 tsp. onion powder

½ tsp. garlic powder

½ tsp. salt

DIRECTIONS

In a medium-sized bowl, combine all ingredients.

Whisk ingredients until fully blended. Adjust seasonings as desired.

BLUEBERRY VINAGARETTE

INGREDIENTS

2 cups blueberries, fresh

2 cups white balsamic vinegar

1 tsp. Stevia

¼ cup honey, raw

3 tbsp. extra-virgin olive oil

½ tsp. salt

½ tsp. pepper

½ tsp. garlic powder

lemon zest

DIRECTIONS

In a medium-sized saucepan, combine blueberries, vinegar, zest, Stevia, and honey. Mix thoroughly, crushing blueberries.

Bring ingredients to a boil and then cover and let simmer on low heat for 15 minutes.

Strain mixture into a bowl and let cool in refrigerator.

Once cool, mix in olive oil, salt, pepper, and garlic powder.

STRAWBERRY DRESSING

INGREDIENTS

1 cup strawberries, organic

1 tbsp. extra-virgin olive oil

½ lemon

2 sprigs rosemary

½ salt

1 pinch pepper, freshly ground

DIRECTIONS

Wash and chop strawberries, removing the stems.

In a food processer combine strawberries, olive oil, rosemary, salt, and pepper. Squeeze lemon juice into the food processor.

Blend until smooth.

LECTIN-FREE CEASAR DRESSING

INGREDIENTS

¾ cup Eden's garbanzo beans

2 cloves garlic

6 tbsp. extra-virgin olive oil

2 tbsp. lemon juice

2 tbsp. nutritional yeast

1 tsp. Dijon mustard

6 drops liquid Stevia

salt

DIRECTIONS

Combine all ingredients in a food processer and blend until smooth. Adjust seasoning as needed. If mixture is too thick, add additional olive oil.

Refrigerate before serving.

Beans

Legumes such as chickpeas should be avoided. However, pressure-cooking legumes can rid them of lectins. If you do not have a pressure-cooker or the time, Eden's brand of legumes is pressure cooked and safe to eat in a low-lectin diet.

ITALIAN-STYLE DRESSING

INGREDIENTS

¾ cup extra-virgin olive oil

¼ white wine vinegar

2 tsp. garlic, freshly chopped

2 tsp. oregano, freshly chopped

1 tsp. basil, dried

½ tsp. onion powder

¼ tsp. lemon juice

1 tsp. parmesan, grated

pepper, freshly ground

salt

DIRECTIONS

Combine all ingredients in a medium-sized bowl and whisk until thoroughly blended. Adjust seasoning as needed.

Transfer mixture to a jar or thoroughly clean squeeze bottle. Shake well before each use.

RANCH-STYLE DRESSING

INGREDIENTS

1 cup goat milk yogurt

1 cup coconut milk

1 tsp. parsley, freshly chopped

1 tsp. dill, freshly chopped

1 tsp. chives, freshly chopped

½ tsp. onion powder

½ tsp. garlic powder

pepper, freshly ground

salt

DIRECTIONS

Combine all ingredients in a medium-sized bowl and whisk until thoroughly blended. Adjust seasoning as needed.

Transfer mixture to a jar or thoroughly clean squeeze bottle. Shake well before each use.

HOMEMADE OLIVE OIL MAYONNAISE

INGREDIENTS

1 egg yolk

1 cup extra-virgin olive oil

1 tbsp. lemon juice, fresh

1 tsp. Dijon mustard

1 tbsp. water

pepper, freshly ground

salt

DIRECTIONS

Combine egg yolk and water into a medium-sized bowl. Whisk together thoroughly.

Add olive oil one drop at a time and whisk the drop completely into the yolk mixture before adding more oil. After a few drops have been completely absorbed into the mixture you may start to add more oil at one time, but slowly.

Once the oil has been completely mixed into the egg mixture add the remaining ingredients until thoroughly mixed.

HONEY MUSTARD DRESSING

INGREDIENTS

¼ cup Dijon mustard

¼ cup of honey, raw

¼ cup of mayonnaise

½ tsp. garlic powder

½ tsp. onion powder

pepper, freshly ground

salt

DIRECTIONS

Combine all ingredients in a medium-sized bowl and whisk until thoroughly blended. Adjust seasoning as needed.

Transfer mixture to a jar or thoroughly clean squeeze bottle. Shake well before each use.

Snacks

The following recipes are the perfect solution to getting you through the afternoon. These small meals are quick and easy to make, as well as portable. They are guaranteed to satisfy your appetite.

SPINACH AVOCADO DIP

Time 10 min | Makes 1 Cup

This low-lectin fresh spinach and avocado dip is a healthy and delicious choice for any party or starter. It's a perfect dip for low-lectin vegetables, such as fresh carrots, radishes, celery, cauliflower, and asparagus.

INGREDIENTS

1 avocado

5 cups fresh spinach

¼ onion, chopped

1-2 cloves garlic

1-2 tbsp. fresh lemon juice

salt

DIRECTIONS

Combine all ingredients in a food processor and blend until thoroughly mixed and thick in consistency.

Add more salt, garlic, lemon juice, or onion until you achieve your desired flavor.

HOMEMADE TZATZIKI DIPPING SAUCE

Time 10 min | Makes 2 cups

This classic Greek dip is low on lectins, but big on flavor. It is also extremely versatile. Use it for dipping vegetables, souvlaki, or as a salad topper.

INGREDIENTS

1 ½ cups goat milk yogurt

½ peeled cucumber

1 tbsp. extra-virgin olive oil

2 cloves garlic

½ lemon

salt

DIRECTIONS

Slowly stir yogurt and olive oil together in a medium-sized mixing bowl.

Add finely minced garlic, lemon juice, and grated cucumber. Add salt to taste.

Refrigerate a few hours before serving.

CUCUMBERS?
While vegetables such as cucumbers and tomatoes are full of lectins, removing the peel and seeds can substantially reduce the lectin content.

Cucumbers are easy to peel and de-seed, making them an easy addition to your diet.

LOW-LECTIN PICO DE GALLO

Time 10 min | Makes 2 cups

This mouthwatering take on a Mexican dish is nightshade free. Consider serving with fish, chicken, and homemade, low-lectin tortillas. It also doubles as a perfect snack.

INGREDIENTS

1 large cucumber, diced

1 cup jicama, diced

½ cup radish, diced

½ cup red onion, diced

½ cup cilantro, chopped

½ tsp. salt

2 tbsp. lime juice

pepper, freshly ground

DIRECTIONS

Peel the skin from both the cucumber and jicama before dicing.

Add cucumber and jicama to the onion, radish, and cilantro in a medium-sized bowl.

Add remaining ingredients and adjust to taste.

SPICY AVOCADO DIP

Time 10 min | Makes 2 cups

This avocado dip is perfect for a low-lectin, afternoon snack. If you prefer it spicier add more onion or cayenne pepper. Try with crispy kale chips!

INGREDIENTS

½ cucumber, diced

½ white onion, medium

¼ bunch cilantro

1 avocado

1 clove garlic

3 tbsp. lime juice

pepper, freshly ground

salt

DIRECTIONS

Peel cucumber before cutting into small pieces. Cut onion into small chunks.

Combine all ingredients in food processer and blend until smooth. Adjust seasoning to taste.

ARTICHOKE HUMMUS

Time 10 min | Makes 2 cups

This low-lectin alternative to chickpea-based hummus is easy to make. Makes a great dip for peeled cucumbers, broccoli, and other low-lectin vegetables.

INGREDIENTS

2 cups artichoke hearts in brine

¼ cup avocado oil

1 clove garlic

2 tbsp. fresh lemon juice

extra-virgin olive oil

DIRECTIONS

Drain artichoke hearts thoroughly. Remove peel from garlic.

Blend artichokes and garlic in food processor. Add remaining ingredients and blend until smooth.

Drizzle with extra-virgin olive oil when serving.

CRISPY OKRA BITES

Time 30 min | Servings 2-4

Not only is this appetizer lectin free, but it is also vegan and gluten free, making it a healthy starter for any meal, as well as a perfect snack at work and in between meals.

INGREDIENTS

12 okra pods

2 tbsp. avocado oil

¼ cup almond flour

¼ cup nutritional yeast

¼ tsp. cayenne pepper

¼ tsp. garlic powder

salt

DIRECTIONS

Preheat oven to 425 degrees Fahrenheit.

In a small-sized mixing bowl, combine almond flour, yeast, cayenne pepper, garlic powder, and salt. Mix and adjust seasonings as desired.

On a cutting board, cut okra pods into slices no thicker than a ½ inch. Move okra slices into a medium-sized mixing bowl and pour in half of the avocado oil, stirring until thoroughly mixed.

Add half the almond flour mix to the sliced okra ensuring that the slices are coated. Pour in the remaining avocado oil and almond flour mix and gently mix together so that each okra slice is as coated as much as possible.

Line a large baking tray with parchment paper and place coated okra slices evenly on top.

Cook for 8-10 minutes before flipping okra slices and cooking for another 8-10 minutes, or until crispy, golden brown.

NUTRITIONAL YEAST
This deactivated yeast has a strong nutty, cheesy, or creamy flavor. For this reason, it is often used as a cheese substitute. It works great in any low-lectin diet.

CRISPY KALE CHIPS

Time 30-40 min | Servings 1-2

These crispy garlic kale chips are the perfect, low-lectin, healthy alternative to potato chips. So go ahead and indulge!

INGREDIENTS

½ bunch kale leaves

½ tbsp. coconut oil

1 tbsp. nutritional yeast

1 tsp. garlic powder

½ tsp. onion powder

salt, preferably sea salt

DIRECTIONS

Preheat oven to 300 degrees Fahrenheit.

Thoroughly wash kale leaves and pat dry with paper towel. Remove stems from kale and use hands to tear into unevenly large pieces.

In a large-sized mixing bowl, combine kale and coconut oil, making sure that the kale is thoroughly coated in oil. Add the remaining ingredients and mix thoroughly.

Line a large baking tray with parchment paper and evenly spread the kale over the tray.

Bake for 10 minutes, after which rotate the pan and bake for another 10-15 minutes.

LOW-LECTIN COLESLAW

Time 1 hour | Servings 8

This creamy coleslaw is packed with lectin-free cabbage, a high source of vitamin K, vitamin C, fiber, and other essential nutrients. Its cheap and easy to make, ensuring it's a great snack and side dish.

INGREDIENTS

½ head of white cabbage

½ head of red cabbage

1 red pepper, peeled

4 oz. homemade mayo

4 oz. gorgonzola

2 tbsp. extra-virgin olive oil

2 tbsp. red wine vinegar

pepper, freshly ground

salt

DIRECTIONS

Cut red pepper into quarters and remove seeds. Carefully peel the outside of each pepper using a peeler. Cut red pepper into thin slices.

Wash cabbage head thoroughly and pat dry with paper towel. Cut in half and shred.

Mix cabbage and red pepper together in a large-sized bowl.

In a medium-sized bowl mix the remaining ingredients until thoroughly mixed.

Add the dressing mixture to the cabbage and stir thoroughly. Liberally season with salt and pepper.

Refrigerate for at least 45 minutes before serving.

TEMPEH FRIES WITH CURRY MAYO DIP

Time 40 min | Servings 6

These delicious tempeh fries are the perfect alternative to nightshade heavy French fries. Paired with a homemade, olive-oil, mayonnaise curry dip, this low-lectin snack will be your new favorite.

INGREDIENTS

16 oz. of grain-free tempeh

5 tbsp. olive oil mayo

2 tbsp. curry powder

½ cup nutritional yeast

4 tbsp. extra-virgin olive oil

pepper, freshly ground

salt

DIRECTIONS

Place tempeh in a large frying pan and fill with enough water so that ¾ of the tempeh block(s) are submerged. Bring to a boil, cover and let simmer until water is evaporated.

Remove tempeh from the frying pan and slice into long pieces.

In a small-sized bowl, mix the nutritional yeast, salt, and pepper. Coat each tempeh slice with the mixture.

In a large frying pan, heat oil over medium-high heat. Fry tempeh strips until both all sides are golden brown. Remove from heat and let drain on paper towel before serving.

Mix mayonnaise and curry powder in a small bowl and put a healthy dollop on each plate with tempeh fries before serving.

AVOCADO FRIES

Time 15 min | Servings 3

These avocado fries are quick and easy to make. Feel freed to add a little cayenne or sriracha to some homemade olive oil mayonnaise for some dip.

INGREDIENTS

3 avocados

1 egg

1 ½ cup almond meal

1 ½ cups extra-virgin olive oil

¼ tsp. cayenne pepper

pepper, freshly ground

salt

DIRECTIONS

In a small-sized mixing bowl, whisk egg until thoroughly beaten.

In another small bowl, mix almond meal, salt, pepper, and cayenne pepper.

Slice and peat each avocado, and peel off the skin. Cut avocado halves into medium-sized vertical strips.

In a large frying pan, heat up olive oil.

Dip each avocado slice in the egg mixture and coat thoroughly in the almond meal mixture.

Cook slices in olive oil until golden brown on all sides. Remove from pan and let drain on paper towel. Cool before serving.

MASHED CAULIFLOWER AND SPINACH

Time 25 min | Servings 6-8

This hearty and healthy dish is the perfect low-lectin snack or side dish. Play around with different vegetables for variety, including kale, sweet potato, and broccoli.

INGREDIENTS

2 cups spinach

1 head cauliflower

½ tsp. garlic powder

1 cup onion, diced

2 tbsp. butter, French

2 tbsp. extra-virgin olive oil

pepper, freshly ground

salt

DIRECTIONS

Cut cauliflower into small florets. Add cauliflower to large pot of boiling water and cook until tender.

In a medium-sized frying pan, heat olive oil over medium heat. Cook diced onions and sauté until clear.

Add spinach to frying pan and cook for 1 minute and remove from heat.

Drain the cauliflower and transfer to food processor. Pulse cauliflower until pureed.

Add the spinach mixture to the food processor, adding the salt, pepper, butter, and garlic powder. Pulse until pureed. If too thick add a tablespoon of water.

Soups & Appetizers

The following recipes are the perfect start to your next dinner party.
Alternatively they work as snacks or small meals in their own right.

SAUTEED GARLIC BUTTER SCALLOPS

Time 15 min | Servings 2-3

These mouth watering garlic butter scallops are a delicious, low-lectin appetizer. Although the recipe calls for a parsley garnish, freshly chopped cilantro would work just as well.

INGREDIENTS

1 lb. fresh, untreated scallops

1 tbsp. extra-virgin olive oil

2 tbsp. butter, melted

¼ cup white wine

3 cloves garlic, minced

½ tsp. cayenne pepper

1 tbsp. fresh parsley, chopped

pepper, freshly ground

salt

DIRECTIONS

Thoroughly wash scallops in cold water and pat them dry with paper towel.

Heat a medium-sized frying pan on medium-high heat, adding the oil and butter once it is heated. Sauté the garlic, then add the scallops and cook until both sides of the scallops turn brown.

Add the remaining ingredients (minus the parsley) and lightly simmer until the scallops are fully cooked.

Sprinkle with freshly chopped parsley for garnish.

CAULIFLOWER LEEK SOUP

Time 30 min | Servings 1-2

Not only is this lectin-free soup perfect for a cold autumn or winter day, it's the perfect alternative to the classic potato leek soup, minus the lectin-loaded tuber.

INGREDIENTS

3 tbsp. extra-virgin olive oil

1 pound leeks

1 head cauliflower

8 cups chicken stock

½ tsp. nutmeg

pepper, freshly ground

salt

Thyme, freshly chopped

Green onion, freshly chopped

DIRECTIONS

Wash leeks and thinly chop. Dice the celery and finely mince the garlic. Wash the cauliflower head and chop into medium-sized florets.

In a large pot, sauté leeks, celery, garlic, cauliflower, nutmeg, salt, and pepper over medium heat. Once leeks are tender, add the stock and cover and let simmer until the cauliflower is tender.

Transfer mixture into a food processer and puree.

Reheat mixture and serve with freshly chopped thyme and green onion.

BROCCOLI, ARUGULA, AND WATERCRESS SOUP

Time 30 min | Servings 2

This easy to make soup is not only low-lectin, but vegan and gluten free. It's a great appetizer for a fall or winter day.

INGREDIENTS

1 tbsp. extra-virgin olive oil

½ yellow onion

1 clove garlic

1 head broccoli

½ cup arugula

¼ cup watercress

pepper, freshly ground

salt

parsley, to garnish

DIRECTIONS

Mince garlic and dice onion. In a medium-sized sauce pan, sauté onions and garlic in olive oil on medium heat until tender.

Wash and cut broccoli into small florets, adding them to the sauce pan. Continue to cook for 5-8 minutes.

Add water and season with salt and freshly ground pepper. Bring mixture to a boil, before turning the heat to low and letting it simmer for 8-10 minutes.

Transfer mixture to a food processer and add the arugula and watercress. Blend until smooth.

Serve soup with a sprig of parsley for garnish.

GARLIC AND THYME ROASTED MUSHROOM CAPS

Time 30 min | Servings 3-4

These savory and mouth watering garlic and thyme roasted mushroom caps are low-lectin and easy to make. Always a crowd pleaser at any dinner party.

INGREDIENTS

15-20 white mushrooms

3 tbsp. extra-virgin olive oil

2 cloves garlic

2 tbsp. butter

½ tsp. garlic powder

2 tbsp. fresh thyme

5 tbsp. parmesan, freshly grated

1 ½ tbsp. lemon juice

pepper, freshly ground

salt

DIRECTIONS

Preheat the oven to 400 degrees Fahrenheit.

Wash mushrooms thoroughly and cut the stalks to an even level. Finely mince the garlic and chop the thyme.

In a medium-sized frying pan on medium-high heat, lightly fry the mushrooms cap-side down for 3-4 minutes in olive oil.

In a large baking tray, arrange mushrooms cap-side down. In a small mixing bowl, combine butter, garlic, thyme, lemon juice, salt, and pepper. Mix together and pour over the top of each mushroom. Sprinkle grated parmesan over mushroom caps.

Place the baking tray in the oven and cook for 15-20 minutes or until golden brown.

GARLIC LIME PRAWN SKEWERS

Time 1.5-2 hours | Servings 4-6

These garlic lime prawn skewers are a perfect summer low-lectin appetizer. If you don't have access to a barbecue grill, you can roast them in the oven just as easily.

INGREDIENTS

1 lb. fresh shrimp, raw

2 tbsp. extra-virgin olive oil

¼ cup cilantro

2-3 cloves garlic, minced

¼ cup lime juice, fresh

pepper, freshly ground

salt

MATERIALS

wooden skewers

DIRECTIONS

In a medium-sized mixing bowl, mix together oil, lime juice, garlic, salt, and pepper. Add the shrimp to the marinade mix and let sit in the refrigerator for 1-5 hours.

After marinating, create skewers by adding 5-6 shrimp per skewer. If barbequing, set to medium heat and grill skewers for about two minutes on each side, basting with the left over marinade as it cooks.

For oven roasting, preheat oven to 450 degrees Fahrenheit. On a large baking tray place skewers and cook for 5-7 minutes.

Once done, garnish with freshly chopped cilantro.

ZESTY SALMON CAKES

WITH GARLIC AIOLI

Time 45 min | Servings 8-10

This low-lectin appetizer is quick and simple to make. The lemon herb aioli adds a tangy flavor to the salmon cakes, making this starter an instant crowd pleaser.

INGREDIENTS

Salmon Cakes

12 oz. salmon, flaked

¼ cup sweet potato, pureed

1 tbsp. parsley, chopped

1 tbsp. Dijon mustard

1 tsp. lemon zest

1 tbsp. lemon juice

3 tbsp. capers, liquid drained

1 medium-sized egg, beaten

3-4 green onions, chopped

pepper, freshly ground

salt

Dressing

1 tbsp. lemon juice, fresh

1 egg yolk

½ tsp. Dijon mustard

½ cup extra-virgin olive oil

2 cloves garlic

1 tbsp. parsley, chopped

1 tsp. dill, chopped

DIRECTIONS

Salmon Cakes

Preheat the oven to 350 degrees Fahrenheit.

In a medium-sized mixing bowl, combine all ingredients, ensuring they are thoroughly mixed.

Take a large baking tray and liberally grease with extra-virgin olive oil.

With a spoon, scoop the mixture into 8-10 patties on the the baking tray, using the back of the spoon to pat down and shape each patty.

Bake for 12-15 minutes in the oven before flipping each patty over and baking for another 12-15 minutes.

Dressing

In a food processor, combine egg yolk, lemon juice, and Dijon. Mix the ingredients until fully blended and *slowly* begin to add the olive oil as you mix.

Mince the garlic and add it to the mixture with the remaining ingredients.

Mix by hand until achieve the desired consistency.

CREAM OF CHICKEN SOUP

Time 80 min | Servings 5

Full of healthy vegetables and protein, this savory soup is the perfect comfort dish. Serve before a full meal or as a standalone meal.

INGREDIENTS

1 lb. chicken breast

1 head cauliflower, chopped

1 white onion, diced

4 stalks celery, chopped

2 cloves garlic, minced

3 leeks, chopped

4 cups chicken broth

1 can coconut milk

3 tbsp. coconut oil

2 ½ tsp. thyme, freshly chopped

2 tsp. parsley, freshly chopped

pepper, freshly ground

salt

green pepper, garnish

DIRECTIONS

Preheat oven to 350 degrees Fahrenheit.

Place chicken breasts in a medium-sized baking dish and add a small layer of chicken broth, salt, and pepper. Cook in oven for 25 minutes or until fully cooked.

Remove chicken from oven and let cool before dicing each breast.

In a large pot, heat coconut oil until melted. Add leeks, onions, and celery, and sauté until tender.

Add cauliflower and garlic and sauté for another 10 minutes.

Add broth, coconut milk, thyme, parsley, salt, and pepper. Bring to a boil and then let simmer without a lid for 25 minutes.

Pour mixture into a food processor and blend until smooth. Return to pot and add diced chicken.

Serve and top with freshly copped green onion and pepper.

COCONUT SHRIMP

Time 25 min | Servings 4-6

These coconut shrimp are the perfect appetizer or snack for when you're in a hurry. Consider garnishing with fresh parsley or cilantro.

INGREDIENTS

1 lb. fresh, raw shrimp

2 eggs

2 cups unsweetened coconut, shredded
coconut oil

pepper, freshly ground

salt

DIRECTIONS

Beat eggs, salt, and pepper together in a medium-sized bowl.

Pour shredded coconut into another bowl.

Peel and rinse shrimp. Dip each shrimp in egg and then shredded coconut, ensuring they are completely coated.

Heat a ½ inch of coconut oil in large frying pan over medium-high heat.

Fry each shrimp until golden brown.

CREAMY BROCCOLI SOUP

Time 15 min | Servings 2-3

This delicious take on cream of broccoli soup is low-lectin and perfect for warming you up on a cold winter day. Feel free to use goat's milk as a substitute for coconut milk.

INGREDIENTS

1 large head broccoli

½ head cauliflower

1 small white onion, diced

2 cups vegetable broth

1 cup coconut milk

½ cup water

pepper, freshly ground

salt

DIRECTIONS

Cut broccoli and cauliflower into small pieces. Place in a large pot.

Add onion, broth, and water to the pot and bring to a boil. Cover with a lid and let simmer over medium heat for 10 minutes.

Remove lid and add coconut milk, salt, and pepper and bring to boil.

Transfer mixture to food processor and blend until smooth.

Heat up before serving.

HEARTY, HEALTHY CHICKEN SOUP

Time 45 min | Servings 4

This take on the classic chicken soup will keep you warm and comfortable on cold days and sick days. Free-range, grass-fed turkey is a great substitute for chicken.

INGREDIENTS

1 lb. chicken breast, diced

2 tbsp. extra-virgin olive oil

1 small white onion, diced

1 carrot

1 tbsp. grated ginger

¼ tsp. cumin powder

½ tsp. chili powder

4 cups chicken stock

1 bunch kale, chopped

pepper, freshly ground

salt

DIRECTIONS

In a medium-sized pot, heat olive oil on medium heat. Add onions and cook until tender and clear.

Place diced chicken breasts in pot and cook until done all the way through.

Add carrots, ginger, cumin, and chili, stirring until thoroughly mixed and continue to cook for another 5 minutes.

Add the chicken stock and bring soup to a boil. Reduce heat and let simmer for another 20-30 minutes. Stir occasionally.

Add chopped kale and cook for another 5 minutes.

Entrees

The following entrees show that a low-lectin diet doesn't need to boring. The versatility of the diet will wow your family and dinner guests. Don't be afraid to substitute different items to keep dinners fresh and exciting.

ROASTED ROSEMARY CHICKEN THIGHS

Time 40 min | Servings 4

A warm, savory dish, grilled rosemary chicken thighs are always a homemade favorite. Consider pairing with grilled asparagus and mushrooms, or fried bok choi.

INGREDIENTS

4 large, boned chicken thighs

1 tbsp. extra-virgin olive oil

2-3 cloves garlic

12 sprigs rosemary

1-2 lemons

pepper, freshly ground

salt

DIRECTIONS

Preheat oven to 450 degrees Fahrenheit.

Finely chop garlic and mix with olive oil and rosemary in a small bowl.

Liberally salt and pepper chicken thighs on both sides. Brush both sides of the chicken thighs with the olive oil mixture.

Place chicken thighs in cooking pan and squeeze fresh lemon juice over the pan.

Roast in the oven until the chicken thighs are cooked through, approximately 30 minutes, flipping the chicken over halfway through.

GRILLED CHICKEN WITH AVOCADO BLUEBERRY SALAD

TOPPED WITH OLIVE OIL AND GOAT CHEESE

Time 40-80 min | Servings 2

As this recipe proves, salads don't have to be boring. This quick, low-lectin salad will leave you feeling fresh and healthy for the rest of the day.

INGREDIENTS

1 large avocado

½ cup blueberries, fresh

2 cups spinach

2-3 radishes

½ cup goat cheese, crumbled

extra-virgin olive oil

oregano, freshly chopped

2 chicken breasts

pepper, freshly ground

salt

Variations:

Consider swapping out grilled chicken for freshly grilled prawns.

Alternatively, go sans meat for a vegetarian option.

DIRECTIONS

Wash and slice radishes into thin horizontal pieces. Fill large salad bowl with a bed of freshly washed spinach. Add radish slices.

Cut avocado in half and remove pit. Using a small knife slice vertical strips of avocado and add to the salad. Sprinkle blueberries and and goat cheese on top. Mix with olive oil, adding salt and pepper as desired.

Preheat the grill to medium-high heat, approximately 400 degrees Fahrenheit.

Take chicken breast and cut breast in half width-wise. Using a meat tenderizer (or rolling pin) pound the thickest parts of the the chicken breast until the entire portion is the same thickness.

Place the chicken breasts in a large bowl and let marinate for up to an hour in oregano, olive oil, salt, and pepper.

Grill chicken for approximately 4 minutes on each side, ensuring that they are no longer pink in the middle before serving.

Place grilled chicken on top of salad and serve.

LOW-LECTIN BEEF CHILI

Time 120 min | Servings 4-6

For those who crave a hot, comforting bowl of chili, this recipe lets you indulge your craving with a low-lectin, beef chili, free from legumes and nightshades.

INGREDIENTS

2 onions, chopped

3-4 cloves garlic

4 stalks celery

1 cup mushrooms, fresh

2 pounds organic beef, ground

½ cup extra-virgin olive oil

3 cups beef stock, low-sodium

1 cup red wine

1 ½ tbsp. ground cumin

2 tbsp. smoked chipotle sauce

1 ½ tsp. garlic powder

1 tsp. onion powder

1 tsp. paprika

pepper, freshly ground

salt

sour cream

green onion

DIRECTIONS

Dice the onions, celery, and mushrooms, before sautéing in a large sauce pan over medium-high heat in half of the olive oil. Add a pinch of salt and stir regularly.

Mince the garlic and add to the mix once the celery is tender. Add the ground beef, spices, chipotle sauce, and the remaining olive oil.

Continue to cook on medium-high heat, stirring occasionally, until the ground beef has browned.

Add the stock and wine and let simmer on low-medium heat for up to 1 hour.

Season with salt and freshly ground pepper to taste. Serve with a dollop of sour cream and chopped green onions.

PISTACHIO CRUSTED SALMON

Time 30 min | Servings 2

This simple and easy to make dish is rich in Omega-3 fatty acids and protein. This delicious, low-lectin dish will go over well with any seafood fan. Best pared with a spinach, arugula medley drizzled with a honey mustard dressing.

INGREDIENTS

2 (6 oz.) wild salmon fillets

1 tbsp. extra-virgin olive oil

¼ cup pistachio nuts

½ lemon

¼ tsp. lemon zest

1 tbsp. Dijon mustard

1 tbsp. raw honey

½ cup grated parmesan

DIRECTIONS

Preheat oven to 375 degrees Fahrenheit.

In a medium-sized mixing bowl, mix lemon juice, lemon zest, honey, and mustard.

Grease a large baking sheet thoroughly with olive oil. Place salmon fillets evenly across sheet.

Thoroughly coat salmon fillets with lemon, honey, and mustard mixture.

In a food processor, combine olive oil and pistachios and pulse until the mixture is coarse.

Spoon the pistachio mixture evenly on top of salmon fillets, pressing lightly with the back of the spoon to spread.

Cook for 15-20 minutes, or until salmon is cooked through and the pistachios are golden brown in color.

GRILLED CHICKEN SOUVLAKI

WITH HOMEMADE TZATZIKI SAUCE

Time 2-4 hours | Servings 6-8

This easy to make low-lectin meal is packed with protein and served with a delicious homemade tzatziki dipping sauce. Serve with a fresh Greek salad, minus the tomatoes, with peeled cucumbers, pitted black olives, sliced red onions, and crumbled goat cheese tossed in extra-virgin olive oil with freshly ground pepper.

INGREDIENTS

3 tbsp. extra-virgin olive oil

6-8 boned chicken thighs

2 lemons

¼ cup white wine

½ tsp. onion powder

½ tsp. basil powder

½ tsp. garlic powder

1 tsp. oregano flakes

pepper, freshly ground

salt

DIRECTIONS

In a large bowl, mix chicken thighs, 1 tbsp. olive oil, freshly squeezed juice from lemons, and white wine.

Stir and mix in onion, basil, garlic, and oregano flakes. Liberally season with salt and freshly ground pepper. Ensure all pieces of chicken are thoroughly coated. Cover and marinate in the fridge for 1-4 hours.

Coat grill or large sauce pan with the rest of the olive oil.

On low-medium heat cook chicken thighs until nicely browned on the outside. Flip the chicken thighs and cook until cooked all the way through.

Remove chicken thighs from heat and let sit for 5-7 minutes before serving.

TOMATO AND NIGHTSHADE FREE MARINARA PASTA SAUCE

Time 120 min | Servings 4-5

High-lectin nightshades such as tomatoes are ubiquitous in our modern diet, but for those looking for a tasty, low-lectin alternative to tomato-based marinara sauce, look no further. This simple to make recipe uses carrots and beets to make a low-sugar, low-lectin alternative the whole family will love. Serve over zucchini noodles or a bowl of freshly chopped kale. Add grilled chicken or prawns if desired.

INGREDIENTS

1 tbsp. extra-virgin olive oil

2 yellow onions

3-4 cloves garlic

1 pound carrots

1 medium-sized beet

1 cup water

1 tsp. oregano flakes

1 tsp. basil flakes

2 lemons

pepper, freshly ground

salt

DIRECTIONS

Dice onions and sauté in a medium-sized sauce pan with olive oil on medium heat. Stir occasionally and cook until onions are clear and tender.

Mince garlic and add to sauce pan. Cook and stir regularly for 1-2 minutes.

Dice the carrots and beets and add to the mixture with the cup of water, bringing the mixture to a boil. Cover and let simmer on low heat for 45 minutes to an hour, or when the beets are fork-tender.

Pour mixture into a food processor, adding salt, ground pepper, oregano, basil, and freshly squeezed lemon juice. Blend until smooth or desired consistency.

BAKED GARLIC CHICKEN
WITH ROASTED ASPARAGUS
Time 40 min | Servings 4-6

Not only is this meal easy to make, it is a guaranteed crowd pleaser. If you're running low on time, this is the perfect, low-lectin dish that will make you and your family ask for seconds. Serve garlic chicken on a bed of Miracle Rice.

INGREDIENTS

4 chicken breasts

4-5 cloves of garlic

1 tbsp. extra-virgin olive oil

2 tbsp. of brown sugar

parsley, thyme, basil, and oregano flakes, as desired

pepper, freshly ground

salt

1 pound of fresh asparagus

3 tbsp. of extra-virgin olive oil

parmesan

DIRECTIONS

Preheat oven to 450 degrees Fahrenheit.

Mince garlic and sauté in small pan with olive oil. Remove garlic and olive oil from the heat and stir in brown sugar, adding herbs as desired.

Liberally season chicken breasts with salt and freshly ground pepper on both sides.

Take a medium-sized baking dish and brush with olive oil. Place chicken in pan and cover with garlic, olive oil, and brown sugar mix. Place pan in oven and cook until chicken is cooked through, approximately 25-30 minutes.

Take a large baking pan and brush liberally with olive oil.

Spread asparagus over the baking pan and coat with olive oil. Bake in the oven for 10-15 minutes at 450 degrees Fahrenheit (for the last 10-15 minutes the chicken is cooing).

Use a fork to determine if the asparagus is tender on the inside. If not, continue baking for another 5 minutes, or until tender. Remove from oven and serve with garlic chicken.

Miracle Rice
Miracle Rice is a low-calorie, gluten-free, lectin-free alternative for basic rice dishes. Made from the root of the konnyaku imo plant, this remarkably healthy substitute is widely available online and in stores.

WILD SALMON WITH CREAMY PESTO SAUCE

Time 20 min | Servings 4

Rich in Omega-3 fatty acids and a great source of protein, grilled salmon is a healthy addition to anyone's diet. The creamy pesto topping is a delicious and savory addition to anyone's low lectin cooking repertoire. Consider serving with an arugula, spinach, and rocket salad medley.

INGREDIENTS

Pan Seared Salmon

4 (6 oz.) wild salmon filets

1 tbsp. extra-virgin olive oil

pepper, freshly ground

salt

Creamy Pesto Sauce

½ cup extra-virgin olive oil

½ cup freshly grated parmesan

⅓ cup pine nuts

3 cloves of garlic

½ cup of goat milk yogurt

pepper, freshly ground

salt

Variations:
Consider using creamy coconut milk instead of goat milk yogurt.

DIRECTIONS

Pan Seared Salmon

Preheat a medium-sized frying pan to medium-high heat.

Brush both sides of salmon fillets with olive oil and liberally season with salt and freshly ground pepper.

Pan sear the salmon fillets in olive oil for approximately 3-4 minutes per side.

Creamy Pesto Sauce

Add garlic to food processor and pulse until coarse in texture.

Add the pine nuts, parmesan, salt, and pepper and blend until the pine nuts are crushed.

Add olive oil and pulse until smooth. You may add more olive oil until you are satisfied with the consistency of the mix.

In a small pan on low-medium heat, warm up the yogurt stirring constantly for 2 minutes. Remove yogurt from heat and add pesto sauce.

Pour creamy pesto sauce over salmon fillets.

TEMPEH CAESAR SALAD

WITH LECTIN-FREE DRESSING

Time 20 min | Servings 4-6

This recipe is a low-lectin, vegetarian alternative to the traditional Caesar salad. Check out our homemade Caesar salad dressing for the perfect topping to your dish.

INGREDIENTS

1 head romaine lettuce, large

6 oz. tempeh, grain-free

2 tbsp. extra-virgin olive oil

2 tbsp. nutritional yeast

¼ tsp. Italian seasoning

pepper, freshly ground

salt

DIRECTIONS

Thoroughly wash romaine lettuce, patting dry with paper towel. Cut lettuce into bite-size pieces and transfer to large-sized mixing bowl.

In a medium-sized pan, place the tempeh and fill the pan up with water until ¾ of the block of tempeh is submerged.

Bring the water to a boil and let sit until it has evaporated. Remove tempeh from pan.

In a small mixing bowl, stir yeast, salt, pepper, and Italian seasoning until thoroughly mixed.

Cut the tempeh into strips. Rub the mixture over all sides of the tempeh strips.

In a medium-sized pan over low heat, cook tempeh strips in olive oil until golden brown.

Pour dressing over romaine lettuce and dish into serving bowls. Top with tempeh strips and serve with freshly ground pepper.

Tempeh
Tempeh is a meat substitute made from cooked and fermented soybeans. While soy in general should be avoided on a low-lectin diet, grain-free tempeh products are included in the 'yes' list of foods to eat.

BASIL PESTO PASTA
WITH LOW-LECTIN ZUCCHINI NOODLES

Time 30 min | Servings 2-4

A healthy addition to any diet, this zucchini noodle (zoodles) basil pesto pasta is a nutritious, gluten free dish that is simple and quick to make. While zucchini does contain some lectins, you can substantially reduce the quantity of lectins by first peeling the zucchini and removing seeds prior to processing the noodles.

INGREDIENTS

Noodles

2 zucchinis

1 tbsp. extra-virgin olive oil

pepper, freshly ground

salt

Basil Pesto Sauce

2 cups basil leaves, chopped

½ cup extra-virgin olive oil

½ cup parmesan, grated

¼ cup pine nuts

3 cloves garlic

pepper, freshly ground

salt

DIRECTIONS

Noodles

Peel outer layer of the zucchinis and remove seeds. Cut length-wise strips of zucchini with a vegetable peeler or grater. You can also use a spiralizer to create more spaghetti-style strips.

On medium heat, warm olive oil in a frying pan. Add zucchini noodles and let simmer for 3-5 minutes, tossing with tongs regularly. Add salt and pepper to taste.

Drain the zucchini noodles in a colander and let sit for 5-10 minutes before serving.

Basil Pesto Sauce

Place garlic in food processor and pulse until coarse in texture. Add the pine nuts, parmesan, salt, and pepper and blend until the pine nuts are crushed.

Wash basil before chopping. Add basil and olive oil to the food processor and pulse until smooth. You may add more olive oil until you are satisfied with the consistency of the mix.

Pour the mixture over your zucchini noodles and grate fresh parmesan on top for garnish.

GARLIC ROASTED CABBAGE WEDGES

Time 40 min | Servings 2-3

This low-lectin vegetarian dish is an easy and quick dish to make when running low on time. Serve with roasted sweet potato slices for a quick, flavorful, meat free, and healthy dinner.

INGREDIENTS

1 head green cabbage

2 tbsp. extra-virgin olive oil

4 cloves garlic

1 tsp. fennel seeds

½ cup parmesan, grated

fresh parsley

pepper, freshly ground

salt

DIRECTIONS

Preheat oven to 400 degrees Fahrenheit.

Finely mince garlic and mix in a small bowl with olive oil, fennel seeds, salt, and pepper.

Cut cabbage into 1-inch-thick slices and arrange on a large baking tray lined with non-stick spray.

Liberally brush both sides of cabbage slices with the olive oil and fennel seed mixture.

Roast in the oven for 15-20 minutes on both sides, or until crispy.

Garnish with sprigs of fresh parsley and grated parmesan.

SALMON BURGERS

Time 60 min | Servings 5-6

These simple, easy to make salmon burgers are packed with Omega-3 fatty acid, antioxidants, proteins, and vitamins. Pair with steamed broccoli and cauliflower garnished with parmesan cheese and miracle rice.

INGREDIENTS

1 lb. wild salmon filets

½ cup parmesan cheese

1 clove garlic, minced

1 ½ tsp. Italian seasoning

1 tbsp. parsley, chopped

1 tsp. paprika

2 eggs, beaten

1/3 cup cauliflower

1 lemon

pepper, freshly ground

salt

DIRECTIONS

Preheat oven to 400 degrees Fahrenheit.

Place salmon filets in steamer and let sit for about 15 minutes until filets are flaky and easy to break apart.

Remove filets and shred into a medium mixing bowl.

Wash cauliflower and cut into small florets. Place in a food processor and puree.

Add cauliflower and remaining ingredients to salmon and mix thoroughly.

Line a baking tray with parchment paper.

Form 5-6 patties with the salmon mixture and place on parchment paper. Cook in oven for 5-10 minutes until golden brown. Flip and cook other side for 5-10 minutes.

Serve with fresh wedges of lemon.

Wild Salmon
Always choose wild salmon over farmed salmon. Farmed salmon is significantly higher in contaminants and less desirable Omega-6 fatty acids.

SPINACH AND CHEESE STUFFED CHICKEN

Time 20 min | Servings 4

These stuffed chicken breasts are the perfect savory dish that everyone will enjoy. Try switching out the parmesan cheese for other Italian or French cheeses to change up flavors.

INGREDIENTS

4 chicken breasts

2 tbsp. extra-virgin olive oil

2 cups spinach

1 cup parmesan cheese

1 tbsp. Italian seasoning

½ cup dry white wine

pepper, freshly ground

salt

DIRECTIONS

Cut length-wise pockets into the side of each chicken breast. Do not cut through to the other side. Liberally salt and pepper both sides of the breasts.

In a medium-size frying pan, heat olive oil over medium heat. Sauté spinach in skillet until wilted.

Mix cheese, spinach, and seasoning in a medium-sized mixing bowl. Stuff the chicken breast with the spinach mixture.

In the frying pan, cook stuffed chicken breasts until golden brown on each side.

Add wine to frying pan and reduce heat to low. Cook for another 5 minutes or until chicken is cooked all the way through.

CREAMY GARLIC PORK CHOPS
WITH ASPARAGUS

Time 30 min | Servings 4-5

These creamy, garlic pork chops will be a big hit with everyone. Pair with grilled asparagus, drizzled in extra-virgin olive oil and parmesan.

INGREDIENTS

4-5 boneless pork chops

1 ½ tbsp. butter

1 ½ cup heavy cream, organic

3 cloves garlic, minced

2 tbsp. almond flour

¾ cup parmesan, grated

1 tbsp. parsley, minced

pepper, freshly ground

salt

DIRECTIONS

Melt butter in a large frying pan over medium heat.

Season each pork chop with liberal amounts of salt and pepper on both sides.

Cook each pork chop on both sides for 5 minutes or until golden brown. Cover with lid and turn off heat. Let pork chops sit for 10 minutes or until fully cooked through.

In another large frying pan, cook garlic over medium heat for 2 minutes. Add flour and cream, bringing mixture to a boil and stirring constantly. Reduce heat and let simmer for 2 minutes.

Add parmesan and parsley and stir until thoroughly mixed.

Add pork chops back to mixture and serve.

SWEET POTATO QUICHE

WITH GOAT CHEESE AND LEEKS

Time 75 min | Servings 8

This savory tart eschews the pastry crust for a low-lectin, sweet potato one. Swap out leeks for kale, broccoli, and parsley.

INGREDIENTS

Crust

2 large sweet potatoes

½ tsp. red pepper flakes

1 egg

pepper, freshly ground

salt

Filling

1 leek, sliced

2 tbsp. butter

8 eggs

¼ cup heavy cream, organic

4 oz. goat cheese

pepper, freshly ground

salt

DIRECTIONS

Crust

Preheat oven to 450 degrees Fahrenheit. Line a 9-inch pie pan with parchment paper and grease with olive oil.

Grate sweet potatoes and squeeze out any excess moisture.

Whisk egg, salt, pepper, and red pepper flakes in a medium-sized mixing bowl. Add grated sweet potato and mix until thoroughly combined. Line bottom and sides of pie pan with sweet potato mixture, pressing down slightly.

Cook for 30 minutes in oven. Remove and set aside to cool.

Filling

Reduce oven heat to 350 degrees Fahrenheit.

In a large frying pan over medium heat, cook leeks with salt and pepper until tender. Let cool.

Whisk eggs, salt, pepper, and cream until thoroughly mixed. Add the leeks and ½ of the goat cheese. Stir and then pour mixture into pie crust. Top with the remaining goat cheese.

Bake for 30 minutes and let cool for 20 minutes before serving.

THAI GREEN CURRY CHICKEN

Time 30 min | Servings 4

This spicy curry can be served over Miracle Rice or on its own. Variations include adding kale and fried grain-free tempeh for a vegetarian version.

INGREDIENTS

1 tbsp. extra-virgin olive oil

1-2 tbsp. green curry paste

3-4 chicken breasts

1 can coconut milk

2 lime leaves

1 tbsp. Stevia

handful green beans

handful asparagus spears

pepper, freshly ground

salt

DIRECTIONS

Cut chicken breasts into length-wise strips. Chop green beans and asparagus spears into 2-inch long strips.

In a large frying pan, preferably a wok, heat olive oil over high heat. Add the green curry paste and stir fry for 2 minutes.

Add coconut milk, lime leaves, and Stevia to the curry paste. Stir well until bring to a boil. Reduce heat and let simmer until the sauce has thickened, approximately 10 minutes.

Add beans and asparagus spears and let simmer for another 5 minutes or until tender. Adjust salt and pepper seasoning to taste.

KALE WITH CRISPY COCONUT TEMPEH

Time 20 min | Servings 4-6

This salad is packed with protein and healthy greens and will leave you feeling healthy and full for the rest of the day.

INGREDIENTS

1 bunch kale leaves

3 green onions, sliced

cilantro leaves

2 limes

1 tbsp. extra-virgin olive oil

1 bulb lemongrass

1 ginger root

½ tsp. Thai green chili

1 tsp. coriander, ground

½ cup full fat coconut milk

2 tbsp. coconut oil

8 oz. tempeh, grain-free

sesame seeds

pepper, freshly ground

salt

DIRECTIONS

Wash kale leaves and pat dry with paper towel. Mix green onion, kale, and 2 handfuls of cilantro leaves in a large salad bowl.

Add olive oil and lime juice to salad and mix thoroughly.

Cut 4 strips of zest off the limes and place in mortar and pestle. Add 4 strips of lemon grass, green chili, and 5 strips of ginger root, coriander, salt, and pepper. Begin pounding the mixture until a paste develops.

Transfer paste to a mixing bowl and add coconut milk and cilantro. Mix thoroughly. Adjust salt and pepper to taste.

In a large frying pan heat coconut oil over medium heat.

Dice tempeh and it to the frying pan with green onions. Stir fry until tempeh is golden brown and crispy. Sprinkle with lime juice.

Pour tempeh mix over salad; toss and sprinkle with sesame seeds.

BUFFALO CHICKEN BROCCOLI BOWLS

WITH CAULIFLOWER RICE

Time 25 min | Servings 4-6

These spicy broccoli, chicken bowls are great for everyone who likes their food a bit spicy. Feel free to experiment with different hot sauces. Sauce from cans of smoked chipotle would also work perfectly.

INGREDIENTS

Cauliflower Rice

1 head cauliflower

1 tbsp. extra-virgin olive oil

pepper, freshly ground

salt

Broccoli Bowls

1 lb. chicken thighs, boneless

1 lb. broccoli

1 tbsp. extra-virgin olive oil

¼ cup sriracha

2 tbsp. butter

pepper, freshly ground

salt

Variations:
Punch up your cauliflower rice with mushrooms.

DIRECTIONS

Cauliflower Rice

Wash and cut cauliflower into small florets. Place florets in food processor and pulse until broken down into rice size pieces.

Sauté cauliflower in olive oil over medium heat until tender. Season with salt and pepper.

Broccoli Bowls

Heat oil in a medium frying pan over medium-high heat.

Combine ingredients in a food processer and blend until smooth. Adjust seasoning as needed. Place skinned and boneless chicken thighs in pan and cook until no longer pink in the center.

Cut broccoli into small florets. Add to pan and cover with lid. Let cook for 10 minutes or until tender. Remove from heat.

In medium-sized bowl whisk melted butter and hot sauce. Pour sauce over chicken and toss to coat evenly.

Serve with cauliflower rice.

HONEY SRIRACHA SESAME CHICKEN CAULIFLOWER

Time 50 min | Servings 4-6

This mouthwatering dish is sure to be a crowd pleaser. Experiment with different flavored hot sauces to keep it fresh and interesting.

INGREDIENTS

1.5 lbs. chicken breasts, diced

1 head cauliflower

2 tbsp. coconut oil

¼ cup coconut aminos

½ cup honey, raw

4 cloves garlic, minced

3 tbsp. sriracha

2 tsp. ginger, minced

2 tsp. onion powder

½ cup water

2 tbsp. arrowroot flour

sesame seeds

scallions, chopped

pepper, freshly ground

salt

DIRECTIONS

Preheat oven to 400 degrees Fahrenheit.

Wash and cut cauliflower into medium-sized florets. Transfer to medium-sized mixing bowl and toss with salt and 1 tbsp. melted coconut oil.

Roast cauliflower in oven for 25 minutes. Remove from heat.

Dice chicken breasts and liberally season with salt and pepper. Heat remaining coconut oil in a large frying pan over medium-high heat. Add chicken and stir occasionally until chicken is cooked through. Remove from heat.

In a small pot, combine honey, garlic, ginger, onion powder, sriracha, and aminos. Bring to a boil and then reduce heat and let simmer. Stir often.

Mix the water and arrowroot powder in a measuring cup. Pour into sriracha pot and bring to a boil again. Lower the heat and let simmer until it thickens.

In a large mixing bowl, stir together chicken, cauliflower, and sauce. Add sesame and chopped scallions for garnish.

Desserts

A low-lectin diet doesn't mean you have to ignore your sweet tooth. There are tons of ways to satisfy

DARK CHOCOLATE ALMOND BUTTER COOKIES

Time 20 min | Servings 20-24

A low-lectin diet doesn't mean you have to give up cookies. These dark chocolate almond butter cookies are low-lectin, low-sugar, and dairy-free treats. As an added bonus they are quick and ridiculously simple to make.

INGREDIENTS

1 cup unsalted almond butter

1 egg

3 oz. dark chocolate, 70 % cocoa

¾ cup Sucant

½ tsp. baking soda

¼ tsp. salt

DIRECTIONS

Preheat oven to 350 degrees Fahrenheit.

Except for the chocolate, combine all ingredients in a medium-sized mixing bowl ensuring they are thoroughly mixed together.

Chop chocolate into small pieces. Add chocolate chunks to mixture.

Using a measuring spoon, scoop approximately tablespoon-sized dollops of the mixture on a large baking tray lined with parchment.

Bake in the oven for 10-12 minutes or until they are golden brown.

Remove from oven and let cool before eating.

RICE PUDDING

Time 45 min | Servings 2-4

This lectin-free rice pudding goes great after any meal. Adding fresh, organic berries, such as raspberries or blueberries, adds not only flavor, but makes the desert look great when served. Consider topping with several mint leaves for garnish as well.

INGREDIENTS

4-5 tbsp. arrowroot powder

2 bags Miracle Rice

3 ½ cup unsweetened coconut milk

1 tsp. butter

1 cup Just Like Sugar

1 tbsp. vanilla extract

1 egg

¼ cup cocoa powder

½ cup raspberries

or blueberries

mint leaves, garnish

DIRECTIONS

Preheat oven to 350 degrees Fahrenheit.

In a colander, pour the Miracle Rice and rinse under running water for up to a minute before setting it aside to drain.

In a small-sized mixing bowl, add a ½ cup of the coconut milk and the arrowroot powder, mixing until the powder has fully dissolved in the milk.

Over medium heat, cook the butter and remaining coconut milk, stirring constantly to break up any lumps. Whisk the egg in small mixing bowl. Add the egg, Just Like Sugar, vanilla extract, and cocoa powder to the Miracle Rice in a large mixing bowl.

Using a tablespoon, scoop the arrowroot-coconut milk mixture in one tablespoon at a time, ensuring you thoroughly mix it in before adding more. Continue to add one tablespoon at a time until you achieve the desired thickness.

In a medium-sized baking dish, grease the insides with butter before pouring in the mixture.

Bake in the preheated oven for 15-20 minutes. Let cool before serving and top with berries and fresh mint.

COCONUT ICE CREAM

Time 60 min | Servings 4

This creamy and smooth coconut ice cream is a wonderful low-lectin alternative to other ice creams on the market. Ensure you use a2 Milk made from grass-fed cows and which is antibiotic and hormone free, as well as rBST and A1 casein protein free. For a crunchy treat consider adding coconut flakes to the mix.

INGREDIENTS

1 cup of A2 milk

1 can of cream of coconut

1 ½ cups heavy cream

1 ½ cups coconut, flaked

MATERIALS

ice cream maker

DIRECTIONS

In a food processor, add the cream of coconut and a2 Milk, ensuring its mixed thoroughly.

Transfer mixture to a medium-sized mixing bowl, stir in heavy cream and coconut flakes (optional).

Pour mixture into an ice cream maker and follow the manufacturer's instructions.

KEY LIME PARFAIT

Time 10 min | Servings 2

This low-lectin dessert is a twist on the classic key lime pie. With creamy avocado, coconut milk, and raw honey, this is a delicious after dinner treat.

INGREDIENTS

1 avocado

¼ cup coconut milk

1 lime

2-3 tbsp. honey, raw

salt

pistachios (optional)

DIRECTIONS

Peel and pit the avocado and juice the lime, collecting the zest as well.

Combine all ingredients into a food processor (minus the pistachios) and blend until smooth.

Serve in small bowls and top with shelled pistachios (optional).

LEMON BREAD WITH A SWEET COCONUT-LEMON GLAZE

Time 60 min | Servings 1 loaf

This lemon bread with sweet coconut-lemon glaze is the perfect, low-lectin dessert. Goes great with after dinner coffee.

INGREDIENTS

Loaf

6 eggs

¼ coconut oil

2 lemons

coconut milk

1/3 cup honey, raw

1/3 cup coconut flour

1 tsp. baking soda

¼ tsp. salt

Glaze

1 tbsp. coconut oil

2 tbsp. honey, raw

2 tbsp. coconut milk

1 lemon

½ tsp. vanilla extract

DIRECTIONS

Loaf

Preheat the oven to 450 degrees Fahrenheit.

With a zester or a grater, zest both lemons. Next, cut both lemons in half and freshly squeeze the juice into a measuring bowl. Add enough coconut milk to the lemon juice to make it equal to 1 cup.

Combine all ingredients into a large mixing bowl and thoroughly mix until well blended.

Take a baking pan and grease it with non-stick spray or oil. Pour mix into the well-greased pan and bake in the oven for 35-45 minutes. The top should be golden brown and the cake should be cooked all the way through.

Remove from oven and let cool.

Glaze

In a large mixing bowl, combine all ingredients and mix thoroughly.

Transfer mixture to a small sauce pan and bring to a simmer over low heat. Remove mixture and let it cool. Once the lemon loaf is done cooking drizzle over the top of the loaf and refrigerate loaf for a minimum of 1 hour before serving.

CHOCOLATE PUDDING

Time 10 min | Servings 4-6

This chocolate pudding is quick and easy to make. Consider topping each pudding with whip cream for an even more decadent low-lectin dessert.

INGREDIENTS

1 cup dark chocolate (72% cocoa), chopped

2 avocados

½ cup cocoa powder, unsweetened

½ cup heavy cream

5-10 drops Stevia

1 tsp. peppermint extract

mint, garnish

DIRECTIONS

Peel and pit the avocados and mash in a medium-sized mixing bowl until smooth.

Melt the chocolate in the microwave and add it, along with the cocoa powder and heavy cream to the avocado.

Transfer the mixture to a food processor and blend until smooth.

Transfer the mixture back to a large-sized mixing bowl, adding the stevia and peppermint extract. Adjust seasonings until you have achieved your desired sweetness.

Serve in small bowls with a mint leaf on top.

DARK CHOCOLATE MILK POPSICLES

Time 3 hours | Servings 4-6

These no-nonsense, easy to make popsicles are low-lectin, vegetarian, and gluten free. They make a perfect after dinner treat, especially on hot summer days.

INGREDIENTS

1 can coconut milk

1/3 cup dark cocoa

2 tbsp. honey, raw

1 tsp. vanilla extract

1 pinch salt

MATERIALS

wooden popsicle sticks

popsicle mold

DIRECTIONS

Combine all ingredients in a food processor and then blend until thoroughly mixed.

If mixture is not sweet enough, add additional raw honey and blend again.

Pour the mixture evenly throughout the popsicle mold. Insert popsicle sticks and put in the freezer for at least 3 hours before serving.

COCONUT BLUEBERRY BARS

Time 40 min | Servings 15

This no bake, low-lectin, gluten free dessert is quick and easy to make. These bars are perfect for after dinner deserts or a snack for when you are on the go.

INGREDIENTS

2 cups blueberries, organic

2 cups creamed coconut

2 tsp. vanilla extract

¼ cup honey, raw

DIRECTIONS

In a food processor, blend all ingredients until smooth.

Line the entire 8x8 baking pan including up and over the sides with parchment paper.

Pour the mixture into the baking pan ensuring it is spread evenly throughout. Using a spatula, gently press down on the mixture.

Cool pan in the fridge for 30 minutes.

Remove pan from the refrigerator and remove the cooled mixture by pulling up on the sides of the parchment paper.

Use a knife to cut into squares or rectangles.

CHOCOLATE CAKE WITH ALMOND BUTTER GLAZE

Time 15 min | Servings 4-6

This lectin-free chocolate cake is sure to be a hit at your next dinner party. Quick and easy to make, it proves that you don't need high-lectin foods to make delicious desserts.

INGREDIENTS

2 tbsp. cocoa powder, unsweetened

2 tbsp. Just Like Sugar

¼ tsp. baking powder

1 egg

1 tbsp. heavy cream

½ tsp. vanilla extract

1 tsp. butter

1 tbsp. almond butter, smooth

DIRECTIONS

In a medium-sized mixing bowl, combine the cocoa powder, Just Like Sugar, and baking powder. Ensure the ingredients are thoroughly mixed.

In another medium-sized bowl, combine the egg, heavy cream, and vanilla extract, mixing the ingredients thoroughly.

Pour the egg and cream mixture into the bowl with the mixed dry ingredients. Mix well.

Take a small, microwave safe bowl and grease it with the butter before pouring in the batter. Microwave for 80 seconds.

Remove and heat almond butter in microwave until liquefied.

Drizzle softened almond butter over the chocolate cake.

Made in the USA
Middletown, DE
29 April 2018